The Precision of Retinoscopy Revisited

with Modern Computerized Methods

Louis S Jagerman MD

ABSTRACT

A 1970 publication described the precision of a group of ophthalmologists in performing repeated refractions by means of retinoscopy on a cohort of selected patients. Given the importance of this topic, a new analysis of a segment of the data was performed, applying current and amended methods, particularly modern computerized statistical methods for the analysis of variance (ANOVA). This revealed previous errors but few substantial changes in the outcomes and conclusions.

The Precision of Retinoscopy Revisited with Modern Computerized Methods

Louis S. Jagerman, MD
May 2014

"Retinoscopy is of great importance in refraction...." Over 40 years ago we [1] published the results of our "studies in refraction," particularly concerned with the "precision of retinoscopy." Complex statistical methods were crucial for arriving at our results and for interpreting our conclusions. At that time—the work was done mostly in 1968 and published in 1970—computers were avidly introduced as statistical tools. However looking back today, our procedures were almost laughingly primitive and ponderous. Once our raw data had been acquired and recorded, we labored many weeks in a large computer lab crammed with bulky equipment on tasks that can now be easily completed in minutes on a laptop.

The 1968-1970 work was funded and supervised by the Neurological and Sensory Disease Control Program, a component of the Division of Chronic Disease Programs of the United States Public Health Service (based in 1970 in Rockville, Maryland). [2] That Program no longer exists, upon reorganization in the USPHS and the National Institutes of Health.

We studied retinoscopic refractions performed by five selected ophthalmologists, labeled A through E, on ten selected healthy patients, numbered 1 through 10; the method is detailed in the cited article, and I have attached copies of key pages in an addendum. The statistical protocol we applied was a newly computerized system for the analysis of variance within and between two complex factors. Our statistical procedures also are described in the 1970 publication, but my goal now, in 2014, is to rework some critical data using only a MacBook Pro computer with MS Excel. (Apple ® OS X version 10.7.5; Microsoft ® Excel for Mac 2011 version 14.2.0.) As I will detail, an omission and an error are apparent in the 1968-1970 statistics, and it is clear now that some steps are actually redundant. Nonetheless these defects do not turn out to be critical, so that I am pleased to report that our main conclusions remain intact.

---

[1] Safir A, Jagerman L, Hyams L, and Philpot J: Studies in Refraction: I. The Precision of Retinoscopy. Arch Ophthalmology **84**: 49-61, July 1970.
[2] The Program's Chief was Clifford H. Cole, MD.

The study analyzed of four features of refraction: Sphere, right eye; sphere, left eye; cylinder, right eye; and cylinder, left eye. We did not study axes of astigmatism in detail, as these data were not essential for our goals, and they needlessly complicated the mathematics. To save space in this article, I will only report my reworking of the data on "sphere, right eye." The other sets of data add no important information and lead to no additional conclusions, but all my work is available upon request.

In this context, "precision" is synonymous with reproducibility. Since our focus was on how *precisely* ophthalmologists perform retinoscopy, we studied the results of two refractions performed by individual ophthalmologists on the same eye of the same patient, given a reasonable time gap between the exams (one to three weeks). The intent was to compare the two refractions by noting any differences between them; i.e., we sought to determine how closely the two measurements of sphere and cylinder of one eye agree. In other words we posed the following key question: If an ophthalmologist using retinoscopy "refracts" a patient today and again in two weeks, how much variation between the two refractions will be found?

Of course we generated hundreds of pairs of measurements. The most expeditious mathematical approach was to subtract the one parameter from its corresponding repetition. For example, on the first encounter ophthalmologist A found +0.50D sphere in the right eye of patient 1, and two weeks later ophthalmologist A found +0.25D in the same eye; the key difference obviously is –0.25, and we labeled each such amount, even when zero, by the letter "d." (Subscripts linked each d to the ophthalmologist, the patient, and the refraction [first or second].) It seemed that a logical appropriate statistical analysis should consist of noting the patterns in all the d's. I emphasize that this approach pitted each measurement against its repetition; we simply compared the two sequential measurements.

It was clear to us even in 1968 that this collection of d's is inadequate for a comprehensive statistical analysis of the measurements. The problem was that an acceptable approach entailed considerations of the variability of the individual ophthalmologist, the variability between the five ophthalmologists, the variability of the individual patient, the variability between the ten patients, the effects of patients' gender, and any interaction between these variabilities. For instance, if a particular ophthalmologist already knew the exact refractive status of a particular patient in lieu performing an impartial *de novo* re-measurement, this aspect of the variability would be disturbed. The doctor's retinoscopic performance would depend on and be influenced by his remembering the patient. Moreover, we appreciated that an assessment of the statistical validity of our other conclusions was essential.

3

To meet these goals an accepted well-known statistical system was applied, *the two-way analysis of variance*, commonly called *Two-Way ANOVA*. [3] Here I will call this system simply ANOVA. We had access to an IBM 360-67 computer, considered to be a technical marvel in 1968, which added elements of excitement and innovation to our work. But a key issue I stress now is this: "Variance" has a definite complicated mathematical definition and composition, and it is *not* simply our "d," the difference between two corresponding measurements. To obtain a variance of the kind required in ANOVA, *each measurement is pitted against the average of the two corresponding measurements.* In formal terminology, our d is a "variation" but it is not a variance. We did not make the distinction consistently in 1968.

Arithmetically our d and its corresponding variance are proportional to each other, so that the same trends are apparent in the two collections of data (all the d's or all the variances), but the correct formalism of ANOVA uses only the latter and does so in a more complicated manner, as I will show. In retrospect the space we devoted to the d's in our past publications was mostly wasted; with respect to ANOVA, it indeed was redundant. However at the time, when computerized processing of ANOVA was a novelty, our approach seemed appropriate.

An additional consideration is now more important than ever: A proper variance must also comply with a certain mathematical structure. This is shown by recalling the above example, wherein the first retinoscopy showed +0.50D and its corresponding repetition showed +0.25. Again, d is −0.25 since we compared the two measurements with each other, *but to apply ANOVA we are forced to compare each measurement against the average of these two values. Moreover, we are required to square the two differences and divide that sum by 2−1.*

These steps are implicit in the general equation

$$s^2 = \frac{\Sigma(x_i - \overline{X})^2}{n-1},$$

where s^2 represents variance. Let me elaborate on the elements in this equation.

[3] Gravetter FJ and Wallnau LB: <u>Statistics for the Behavioral Sciences</u>, 9th Edition. Chapters 13-15. Independence, KY 41051. ISBN-10: 1111835764. 2012.

The reason for the label "s²" is that here variance is actually the square root of the standard deviation of the sample. The x_i symbolizes measurements, and since we worked with pairs, the subscript was 1 or 2. The $\bar{X}$ stands for the mean (the average) of the two measurements; in this example the mean (0.50 + 0.25)/2 is 0.375. The comparisons between each measurement and the mean are represented by the minus signs. Moreover these differences are squared. The n is the size of the sample, in this case 2, and the equation calls for subtracting 1. (When the variance of a population rather than a sample is calculated, subtracting 1 from n is not done.)

With the amounts in the example (representing one sample) inserted into this equation we obtain

$$s^2 = Variance = \frac{(0.50-0.375)^2+(0.25-0.375)^2}{1}.$$

The result is that the variance is 0.03125, clearly different from the variation d, −0.25, and I stress again that only the former has a role in ANOVA.

Despite the complexity of variances, these are easy to calculate with a spreadsheet such as Excel, and ANOVA modules are available to automate the entire process. (Incidentally, many dedicated [often cost-free] ANOVA programs are available on-line, so that even access to a spreadsheet is not essential. The remaining issues are deciding on the settings for data organization, and entering the data itself. Of course such capabilities were in the distant future in 1968.)

The primary features of ANOVA, essential in this study, are that it clearly elucidates the variance for ophthalmologists, it separates this from the variance for patients, and it reveals spurious statistical interactions between the performances of ophthalmologists and patients. Thus the end product of ANOVA includes three values, called "computed F statistics" or "computed F-values." In this study (of 2014) the first F-value expresses the variance for ophthalmologists, the second expresses the variance for patients, and the third expresses interactions between the two groups. In each case—and this was not done in 1968, constituting a serious omission—the "computed" F-value is compared against a "critical" F-value obtained from a table or program appropriate to the circumstances. I will present these outputs later in this article.

The next section is primarily procedural and dwells on statistical/mathematical manipulations. It may not be of interest to all readers; please feel to skip to the paragraph beginning with "This ends the procedural section..." on page 12. Here is the situation: In order to arrive at the three computed F-values, a set of intricate mathematical steps is required (rudimentary for modern software) which are summarized in several key equations. To appreciate these equations, we should know that several values in ANOVA are called "sums of squares," obviously where squared values are added up; these are "SS" values identified with subscripted descriptions (o-p interaction means ophthalmologist-patient interaction).

Here are these equations, solvable for the pertinent SS values. (Some terms reflect the custom to arrange the data into tables with rows and columns, which we followed in 1968-1970 and I did again in 2014.)

I show the list of key equations in its entirety on one page to allow a clearer overview. Please note that the second equation has a reference to a footnote.

$$SS_{total} = \Sigma X^2 - \frac{(\Sigma X)^2}{N}$$

$$SS_{total} = SS_{within} + SS_{between} \quad ^{4 \text{ (a footnote, not an exponent)}}$$

or rearranged,

$$SS_{within} = SS_{total} - SS_{between}$$

$$SS_{ophthal} = \Sigma \frac{(\Sigma \text{ for each column})^2}{n \text{ for each column}} - \frac{(\Sigma X)^2}{N}$$

$$SS_{patient} = \Sigma \frac{(\Sigma \text{ for each row})^2}{n \text{ for each row}} - \frac{(\Sigma X)^2}{N}$$

$$SS_{between} = SS_{ophthal} + SS_{patient} + SS_{o-p \text{ interact}}$$

or rearranged,

$$SS_{o-p \text{ interact}} = SS_{between} - SS_{ophthal} - SS_{patient}$$

$$SS_{between} = \frac{(\Sigma X_1)^2}{n_1} + \frac{(\Sigma X_2)^2}{n_2} + \cdots + \frac{(\Sigma X_{rc})^2}{n_{rc}} - \frac{(\Sigma X)^2}{N}$$

---

[4] The equation $SS_{total} = SS_{within} + SS_{between}$ expresses a basic concept in ANOVA: The total variance is the sum of the variance within the variables plus the variance between the variables. In principle, the total is a sum of its parts.
Furthermore, as the subsequent equation $SS_{between} = SS_{ophthal} + SS_{patient} + SS_{o-p \text{ interact}}$ shows, the variance between variables is the sum of three subsidiary variances.

As I indicated, the strategy behind these equations is to start with the total variance in the entire study and to separate or "tease out" the variances of practical interest, namely *the variance for the five ophthalmologists, the variance for the ten patients, and any interactions.* To achieve this goal—i.e. to solve the above equations—the raw data—the measurements—must be manipulated by a combination of adding and squaring carefully selected groups of measurements in proper sequence. Since these groups will contain unequal numbers of elements (e.g., data on 5 ophthalmologists vs. data on 10 patients), some of the SS-values will be divided by "degrees of freedom" based on the group size. These steps, done on $SS_{ophthal}$, $SS_{patient}$ and $SS_{o-p\ interact}$, will yield the three corresponding important calculated F-values.

The 1968-1970 calculations included an error (incorrect addition) in the SS_{total}; 175.832 should have been 171.337. However, this did not affect the rest of the mathematics, and it does not alter the statistical conclusions. The past calculations also include an error in the obtaining the F-value for ophthalmologists (the denominator and numerator were reversed); it should be 1.303 rather than 0.768, but the corrected value is still less than the critical F-value, 3.633, so that again the statistical conclusion is unaffected. In retrospect it is clear that we made serious math mistakes, but we were fortunate that these were not critical and did not lead us to erroneous final conclusions. Of course these errors would have been avoided if today's full computerization had been available.

Let us look at the raw data, keeping in mind that this (2014) article is restricted to the sphere measurements on right eyes, whereas the 1970 publication included all measurements for both eyes. Each of the 50 boxes is a "cell" and a "sample," and each holds the results of the two retinoscopic refractions done one to three weeks apart on a particular patient by a particular ophthalmologist.

The following table (next page) holds the values (variables) inserted into the equations on the previous pages for modern ANOVA statistical analysis. The measurements (in diopters) are shown in equations by the X's.

All Measurements of sphere OD (in diopters) - Cells - Samples

Patients	Ophthalmologists				
	A	B	C	D	E
1	0.50	0.25	0.50	0.00	0.00
	0.75	0.50	0.75	0.50	0.00
2	-1.25	-1.50	-1.50	-1.25	-1.25
	-0.75	-1.25	-1.00	-1.25	-1.25
3	-2.75	-1.75	-2.25	-2.00	-2.00
	-2.75	-1.50	-2.00	-1.75	-1.75
4	0.50	1.25	0.75	1.00	1.00
	1.50	1.25	1.00	1.25	1.00
5	-0.50	0.00	-0.25	0.00	0.00
	0.00	0.00	-0.25	0.00	0.25
6	-1.75	-1.75	-1.75	-2.25	-1.50
	-1.50	-1.25	-1.50	-1.75	-1.50
7	-0.50	0.25	-0.50	0.00	0.50
	0.50	0.25	0.00	0.00	0.50
8	0.50	0.25	0.25	-0.50	0.00
	1.00	0.50	0.75	0.00	0.25
9	-2.50	-2.50	-2.50	-2.75	-2.50
	-1.25	-2.25	-1.50	-2.50	-2.00
10	-3.00	-3.00	-3.00	-3.00	-2.75
	-3.00	-3.00	-2.75	-2.75	-2.50

8

Now the above-mentioned manipulations can be presented. The next logical step is to square every measurement. Each cell thus houses two X^2's.

Squares of all measurements

0.25	0.0625	0.25	0	0
0.5625	0.25	0.5625	0.25	0
1.5625	2.25	2.25	1.5625	1.5625
0.5625	1.5625	1	1.5625	1.5625
7.5625	3.0625	5.0625	4	4
7.5625	2.25	4	3.0625	3.0625
0.25	1.5625	0.5625	1	1
2.25	1.5625	1	1.5625	1
0.25	0	0.0625	0	0
0	0	0.0625	0	0.0625
3.0625	3.0625	3.0625	5.0625	2.25
2.25	1.5625	2.25	3.0625	2.25
0.25	0.0625	0.25	0	0.25
0.25	0.0625	0	0	0.25
0.25	0.0625	0.0625	0.25	0
1	0.25	0.5625	0	0.0625
6.25	6.25	6.25	7.5625	6.25
1.5625	5.0625	2.25	6.25	4
9	9	9	9	7.5625
9	9	7.5625	7.5625	6.25

Sum of all above values is 239.8123.

When all values in this table (the measurements squared) are added together, the sum is ΣX^2, which is 239.8125. This becomes the first term in the right side of the first equation of the above list,

$$SS_{total} = \Sigma X^2 - \frac{(\Sigma X)^2}{N}.$$

Since this form of the equation for SS_{total} has simple terms and lends itself to a numerical solution, it is called the computational version. Of course retinoscopy to 1/1000th (four decimal places) is clinically meaningless, but this is needed for the statistical computations.

The raw data can also be manipulated by adding the two measurements together in each cell (in each sample). Each cell thus houses a Σx.

Totals of cells (samples)

						Row sums
1	1.25	0.75	1.25	0.50	0.00	3.75
2	-2.00	-2.75	-2.50	-2.50	-2.50	-12.25
3	-5.50	-3.25	-4.25	-3.75	-3.75	-20.50
4	2.00	2.50	1.75	2.25	2.00	10.50
5	-0.50	0.00	-0.50	0.00	0.25	-0.75
6	-3.25	-3.00	-3.25	-4.00	-3.00	-16.50
7	0.00	0.50	-0.50	0.00	1.00	1.00
8	1.50	0.75	1.00	-0.50	0.25	3.00
9	-3.75	-4.75	-4.00	-5.25	-4.50	-22.25
10	-6.00	-6.00	-5.75	-5.75	-5.25	-28.75
Column sums	-16.25	-15.25	-16.75	-19.00	-15.50	-82.75

In this and the next table, the value in the right lower corner is a grand total, obtained by adding all row sums or all column sums.

This table provides several useful values: the sum of each row (data on the 10 patients), the sum of each column (data on the 5 ophthalmologists), and a grand total, −82.75, which is the same whether computed vertically or horizontally, as it should be. This grand total, when squared, becomes $(\Sigma X)^2$, equaling 6847.5625.

Meanwhile, the total number of measurements, N, is 100, and $(\Sigma X)^2/100$ is the second term in the right side of the equation,

$$SS_{total} = \Sigma X^2 - \frac{(\Sigma X)^2}{N}.$$

In this manner this equation, the first in the above list, has been solved. It turns out that $SS_{total} = 171.337$, which is the total variance in the entire study. (In 1970 we came up with 175.832.)

I show next how the variance for the ophthalmologists, $SS_{ophthal}$, can be separated or "teased out" of the above total variance; i.e., how can this equation be solved:

$$SS_{ophthal} = \Sigma \frac{(\Sigma \: for \: each \: column)^2}{n \: for \: each \: column} - \frac{(\Sigma X)^2}{N}.$$

The approach is intuitively clear: The above table shows column sums, each column has data on one ophthalmologist, and the second term has already been calculated. Here n is 20 since each column represents 20 measurements. Though the process is tedious and error-prone without a computer program, it turns out that $SS_{ophthal}$ is still 0.446250 when obtained with modern tools.

Here the concept of "degrees of freedom" enters the picture, although this term stems from other procedures in mathematics. The degrees of freedom for the total study is 99 (N=100 but if 99 are known, the last is determined and therefore has "no freedom."). For the 5 ophthalmologists it is only 4. In is important to note that this inequality in group-size must be considered to obtain the correct F-value for the ophthalmologists, and the degrees of freedom for each group allow compensations for their unequal composition. Hence degrees of freedom are a major consideration in ANOVA.

The procedure is revealed in the ratio

$$\frac{SS_{ophthal}}{Degrees \: of \: freedom_{ophthal}},$$

which in this instance is 0.44625/4. The result is 0.1115625, labeled $MS_{ophthal}$ in compliance with the ANOVA system.

A complicating issue arises now, represented in the equations

$$SS_{total} = SS_{within} + SS_{between}$$

or, rearranged,

$$SS_{within} = SS_{total} - SS_{between}.$$

Clearly the total variance is actually the sum of two components. One is SS_{within}, representing variance within the cells or samples, and this is of interest here. The other is $SS_{between}$, representing variance between the cells or samples, and this value alone is of no direct interest here. (In other cases, variance between samples may be crucial. For example, a difference between male and female subjects might be of interest; does gender interfere with the results?)

The former, SS$_{within}$, can be obtained two ways, one of which is directly from the raw data cell by cell (sample by sample); we did just that in 1968, as I will recreate shortly. The second less direct way is by solving the complicated equation for obtaining SS$_{between}$ (the last in the master list) and subtracting the result from SS$_{total}$. Indeed I used both methods in 2014 to check that the outcome is the same, as it should be, but I omit this detail here.

The former direct procedure calls for the next table, wherein the variance is calculated for every cell (sample) using the formal general equation

$$s^2 = \frac{\Sigma(x_i - \bar{X})^2}{n-1}.$$

Cell Variances (within sample variances)

						Row sums
1	0.03125	0.03125	0.03125	0.12500	0.00000	0.21875
2	0.12500	0.03125	0.12500	0.00000	0.00000	0.28125
3	0.00000	0.03125	0.03125	0.03125	0.03125	0.12500
4	0.50000	0.00000	0.03125	0.03125	0.00000	0.56250
5	0.12500	0.00000	0.00000	0.00000	0.03125	0.15625
6	0.03125	0.12500	0.03125	0.12500	0.00000	0.31250
7	0.50000	0.00000	0.12500	0.00000	0.00000	0.62500
8	0.12500	0.03125	0.12500	0.12500	0.03125	0.43750
9	0.78125	0.03125	0.50000	0.03125	0.12500	1.46875
10	0.00000	0.00000	0.03125	0.03125	0.03125	0.09375
Column sums	2.21875	0.28125	1.03125	0.50000	0.25000	4.28125

The lower right corner, 4.28125, is another grand total and represents the variance within the samples, SS$_{within}$. This quantity reflects "interference;" in this case it is a potential tendency of the ophthalmologists' measurement to be swayed by which subject is being measured.

12

Here the concept of "degrees of freedom" reenters the picture: To obtain SS_{within}, only 50 cells were considered, so that the "mean square" for SS_{within} is 4.28125/50 or 0.085625. In the ANOVA system, this value is labeled MS_{within}.

At this point the F-value for ophthalmologists can be calculated, simply from the ratio $MS_{ophthal}$ over MS_{within}. In this case, 0.1115625/0.085625 = 1.30. *This is the calculated F-value representing the variance for the ophthalmologists; it assesses the reproducibility in their performance of retinoscopy. In effect it measures the precision.*

As for the question of variance for patients—how precise are they when re-refracted—the procedures for obtaining $SS_{patient}$, $MS_{patient}$, and the corresponding F-value are similar, save for use of the equation

$$SS_{patient} = \Sigma \frac{(\Sigma\ for\ each\ row)^2}{n\ for\ each\ row} - \frac{(\Sigma X)^2}{N}.$$

Now only *row data* is taken from the same "totals of cells (samples)" table. The n is 10 rather than 20, and the degrees of freedom are 9. Thus $SS_{patient}$ and $MS_{patient}$ turn out to be 161.430 and 17.997 respectively, with the corresponding F-value calculated to be 209.480.

As for interference, the standard method for finding $SS_{o\text{-}p\ interact}$ is via subtraction in the equation

$$SS_{o-p\ interact} = SS_{between} - SS_{ophthal} - SS_{patient},$$

since all three component values are available. The degrees of freedom are 36 (4 by 9), reflecting the two sets of participants. Here the statistics turn out to be 5.179 for $SS_{o\text{-}p\ interact}$, 0.144 for $MS_{o\text{-}p\ interact}$, and 1.680 for the calculated F-value.

This ends the procedural section for my work of 2014.

What remains is to look up the critical F-value in a standard table, *which was not done in 1968*. If performed manually, two items of information are needed for this step: (a) the desired level of confidence—i.e., the probability for erring in our conclusions (the probability of rejecting a null hypothesis that in fact is true), customarily set at 0.05 or less—and (b) the degrees of freedom for the two main variances, here 4 and 9. Modern computerized ANOVA software can provide the critical F-value automatically, and it can even show the actual level of confidence (the p-value) used to judge whether a null hypothesis should be accepted or not.

13

In this case the critical F-value turns out to be 3.633. The entire set of final values can be summarized in an ANOVA table, akin to the one presented in 1970 but with the corrections and additions in the re-analysis of 2014:

Analysis of variance (two-way ANOVA) for spherical repeated retinoscopy by five ophthalmologists on the right eyes of ten patients

Source of variance	SS's	Degr's of freedom	MS's	F-values
Ophthalmologists	0.446250	4	0.111563	1.302920
Patients	161.430625	9	17.936736	209.48013
Interaction	5.178750	36	0.143854	1.680049
Retinoscopies within samples	4.281250	50	0.085625	
Total	171.336875	99		
(Between samples)	(167.055625)	(49)	Critical F	3.633

The last column is the most important, though by convention the entire table is presented in publications. In brief, here is what the F-values tell us:

Ophthalmologists appear precise; two separate retinoscopies are bound to be similar.

Patients appear imprecise; repeated retinoscopies are bound to differ in a patient.

Interaction is negligible; the protocol succeeded in avoiding significant bias from participants influencing each other. This indicates that retinoscopy can be performed objectively.

Incidentally, in scientific research the perm "precise" is akin to the term "reliable;" when they are precise or reliable, repeated measurements are consistent. In contrast, the terms accuracy and validity indicate that a measurement reflects reality; in this case we assumed that retinoscopy actually measures the dioptric state (the refractive state) of the eye. As suggested by its very title, this study focuses on the former, and indeed the reliability of refraction has been examined by others. [5]

---

[5] For instance, Thibos, L. N. et al. Accuracy and Precision of Objective Refraction... Journal of Vision, April 23, 2004 vol. 4 no. 4 article 9

14

Let me elaborate now on the 2014 findings, as was not done in this manner in the past:

Since the computed F for *ophthalmologists* is less than the critical F, we say with a specific degree of certainty, here 95%, that there is no statistically significant variance between ophthalmologists. In customary statistical terminology this inference is also said to be the "null hypothesis," and in this instance the null hypothesis cannot be refuted. *This indeed was also our conclusion less formally and less rigorously in 1968, and it is my conclusion now using the standard ANOVA system: Ophthalmologists appear to be significantly precise in retinoscopy; they tend to find similar results on different occasions; their results appear to be adequately reproducible.*

If the computed F for *patients* were less than the critical F, we could say, with 95% certainty, that there is no statistically significant variance between patients. This inference is also said to be a "null hypothesis;" i.e. the null hypothesis could not be refuted. *This was **not** our conclusion in 1968 and it is **not** mine now, despite using the standard ANOVA system: patients appear to be significantly imprecise in undergoing retinoscopy; they tend to yield different results on different occasions; their cooperation appears to be inadequately reproducible.* The issue of imprecision among subjects, even selected ones, was not explored further in this study, but as experienced refractionists will attest, it can be a serious clinical problem.

Since the computed F for *interaction* is less than the critical F, we say, with 95% certainty, that there is no statistically significant interaction between ophthalmologists and patients. This inference is also said to be a "null hypothesis;" i.e. the null hypothesis regarding interactions cannot be refuted. *This indeed was our conclusion in 1968 and it is mine now: ophthalmologists appear to perform retinoscopy on different patients objectively and without significant bias, and (incidentally) patients appear to respond without significant bias to different ophthalmologists.* In particular and more importantly, no evidence was found to indicate that the ophthalmologists' second measurement on a given patient was tainted by his recalling, remembering or "peeking" at the result of first measurement. (By means of shielding and other provisions, we ensured that the ophthalmologist could not identify the subject during the examination, and the records of past results were not revealed to the ophthalmologists. Patients could see the ophthalmologist, but apparently this did not affect their cooperation.)

At this juncture I should repeat that I see no purpose now in reporting the reworking the statistics regarding the other main aspect of retinoscopy, namely the measurement of astigmatism. The 1970 paper covers this aspect, but the effort would require many pages of even more tedious mathematics, and a skeletal investigation shows that no additional conclusions would be uncovered.

In 1970 we recognized that estimating the precision of gauging cylinder axis is a different problem that is not relevant for our study, and the statistical approach would also be quite different. Indeed a separate mathematical approach would be required. For instance, we would have to accommodate the facts that a zero cylinder axis does not indicate zero astigmatism, and that an axis of, say, 40 degrees does not mean that the astigmatism is "twice as bad" as 20-degree astigmatism.

In 1970 we also reported several ancillary but interesting inferences gleaned from our results. The same inferences are justified today. For example, although all five ophthalmologists knew they were being rated and were remarkably consistent, they differed somewhat from each other in their precision, even with regard to which eye, right or left, they were refracting. Similarly, although all patients were deemed to be healthy and cooperative, some were substantially better than others at allowing accurate retinoscopy, and refractionists should be aware of this factor. We are reminded that refraction and retinoscopy are an art that entails a complex interaction between two human beings!

On the other hand we openly acknowledged in 1970, as I do again now, that this study is in many ways exceptional and atypical of how refraction and retinoscopy are performed "in the real world." Not only were we selective in whom we accepted as subjects, but the design was extremely selective in who was chosen to perform the measurements: five co-operative ophthalmologists, each highly motivated and obviously interested in gaining insights into refraction and retinoscopy. Moreover repeated examinations were essential to the study, as is unusual in a clinical setting.

For example we were sharply questioned by our critics as to whether the study would have been accepted by a major ophthalmic journal—or even supported by an agency of the US Public Health Service—had our data shown that retinoscopic repeated examinations by ophthalmologists are statistically *not* reliable or precise! Since I was the youngest of the five ophthalmologists, I was even asked whether I would have allowed public dissemination of the conclusion that my retinoscopic skills were questionable.

By coincidence, we were also working on a prototype of an automatic retinoscope, and years later sophisticated and refined models have helped in this area. On the other hand we should keep in mind that in the usual setting retinoscopy is only one component of refraction.

I conclude that an updated and refocused 2014 reworking of our 1968-1970 study yields largely the same equally valid outcomes, despite some errors, omissions, and extraneous steps. Ophthalmologists are quite precise and can be objective in performing retinoscopy. However, patients are significantly less precise.

Addendum I:

We assumed that readers are trained and experienced refractionists who require no explanation of the nature and performance of retinoscopy. However, here I insert a very brief review: Visible objects reflect or emit light. Ideal visual acuity requires that rays of light from such objects be sharply focused onto the retina. For example the essentially parallel rays of light from a distant object ideally should converge on one small region of the retina, and there they should form a clear image. However the reverse is also true: If the retina could emit light, the ideal eye is such that the emitted rays of light are parallel. Fortunately, the human retina is somewhat reflective, so that when it is illuminated it acts as a source of light.

In retinoscopy, the retina is illuminated through the pupil by an external source of light, so that rays of light, reflected from the retina, exit the eye through the pupil. The retinoscopist then determines whether the exiting rays of light are parallel. If they are not, the retinoscopist places certain lenses in front of the eye (where glasses would be located) that make the exiting rays parallel. If the exiting rays are not parallel but convergent, the eye is nearsighted (myopic), and if they are divergent, the eye is farsighted (hyperopic). Astigmatism complicates this principle, because in the presence of astigmatism the vergence is different in different meridians. (These meridians can be thought of as compass directions.)

The dioptric "power" of the lens or combination of lenses required to parallelize the exiting rays of light identifies the refractive state of the eye – nearsightedness, farsightedness and/or astigmatism. In short, the retinoscopist determines which lens or lenses make exiting rays parallel. The main challenging aspect of retinoscopy—the one requiring the most skill—is for the retinoscopist to judge when the exiting rays of light have been made parallel.

Incidentally, the same principles have been applied and greatly refined in the design of modern "automatic" retinoscopes, wherein different kinds of light (infrared, certain LASER's) illuminate the retina, and the exiting light is analyzed in the form of many thin beams to yield a mosaic-like composite of many "mini-retinoscopies." I describe the optics, math and practical applications in a separate book. [6]

Addendum II:

For readers wishing to see the most important pages of the 1970 paper, a copy (courtesy of Archives of Ophthalmology) of the first few pages is attached. The resolution is poor, as original prints are no longer available and the supplies of reprints have been exhausted.

---

[6] Jagerman, L. S. Ophthalmologists, Meet Zernike and Fourier! Trafford Publishing, Victoria, Canada, 2007. (Available at Amazon.com.)

Studies in Refraction

I. The Precision of Retinoscopy

Aran Safir, MD, New York; Louis S. Jagerman, MD;
John Philpot, PhD, New Brunswick, NJ; and
Lyon Hyams, MD, Arlington, Va.

A clinical study was done to determine how precisely ophthalmologists perform retinoscopy. Ten subjects were examined by five ophthalmologists on two separate occasions. Statistical analysis of the results showed that the physicians' precision was unaffected by patients' sex or type of refractive error; the physicians in general agreed in their estimates of the magnitudes of the refractive errors, but their precision varied significantly; cylinder power was measured more precisely than sphere power; and right eyes were measured more precisely than left eyes. Quantitative estimates are given for the variability of replicate retinoscopic measurements. Suggestions are made for techniques of clinical retinoscopy which may minimize certain errors.

RETINOSCOPY is of great importance in refraction, perhaps more in the United States than elsewhere. For many practitioners it is the foundation stone of their refraction procedure, a test which they have mastered after long effort, and to whose employment they devote much time. Therapeutic judgments, patients' comfort and welfare, and the expenditure of large sums of money for eyeglasses may be based on the practitioner's skill in retinoscopy. Yet little effort has been made to determine how good this procedure is and how well practitioners perform it.

Retinoscopy is of equal, if not greater, importance to researchers in refraction, for it is almost the only objective method of refraction that has been found applicable to the evaluation of statistical samples of patients in the study of incidences and prevalences of refractive errors, and the effects of drugs and therapies on the refractive state of the eye.

In all the uses of retinoscopy, both in practice and in investigation, we make measurements whose accuracy and precision are subject to uncertainty. It is impossible for a practitioner or a researcher to know in any given case how much of the variability of refractive error he is measuring is due to the variability of the refractive error itself, and how much of it is due to the variability of the method of measurement. It is our purpose in this series of papers, of which this is the first, to analyze some of the sources of uncertainty and error in the measurement of refraction so that practitioners and researchers may better judge the reliability of their findings.

There have been some attempts to evaluate the worth of retinoscopy. Volk,[1] evaluating an optometer (Rodenstock), made a quantitative comparison of his retinoscopy and the patients' subjective refraction. Since there was only one refractionist and no true replication of data, the conclusions were limited in their scope. Freeman and Hodd[2] used replications, but they compared retinoscopy done by one refractionist with subjective refractions done on the same subjects by another refractionist. Their conclusions are therefore limited to comparisons of the abilities of two individual practitioners using different methods.

Hirsch[3] made a better approach to the problem by recording replicate retinoscopic measurements. Unfortunately, he made no record of the identities of the examiners, so that his data and conclusions are partially inferential. He did, however, present some clear statements of the dilemma regarding

Submitted for publication Dec 29, 1969.

From the Department of Ophthalmology, Mount Sinai School of Medicine, New York (Dr. Safir); Division of Biostatistics, Department of Community Medicine, Rutgers Medical School (Dr. Jagerman), and Center for Computer and Information Services, Rutgers, the State University (Dr. Philpot), New Brunswick, NJ; and the Neurological & Sensory Disease Control Program, Public Health Service, Arlington, Va.

Reprint requests to Department of Ophthalmology, Mount Sinai School of Medicine, Fifth Ave and 100th St, New York 10029 (Dr. Safir).

confidence in measurements and some firm evidence that repeat-retinoscopies, done on the same individual, may vary by rather large amounts.

The purpose of this report is to describe an experiment which we performed in order to determine the precision of retinoscopic measurement of the refractive error of the eye. Precision, the ability to duplicate a measurement, must be distinguished from accuracy. Accuracy (also called validity) gives information on how closely the measurement approaches the true value of the quantity sought. So, for example, if a patient's true refractive error is 3 diopters and, each of three times measured, it is recorded by the refractionist as 2.00 D ± 0.25 D, then this refractionist demonstrates better precision than accuracy.

Precision (often called reliability) must be more clearly defined before we can discuss it meaningfully. It is too general merely to state that precision is the ability to reproduce a measurement. The variable measured, the circumstances of measurement, the person measuring, and the subjects measured must be specified.

In our experiments, we consider five aspects of the reliability of retinoscopic measurement. These can best be presented in the form of questions.

1. To what degree can refractionists, in general, duplicate their retinoscopy with subjects, in general? We will call this *general replicability*.

2. Is the replication error the same for different subjects, or do the examinations of some subjects by the "average" ophthalmologist yield a greater variation than the examinations of other subjects? We will call this the *subject variability of replication*.

3. Is the replication error the same for different ophthalmologists, or does the retinoscopy of the "average" patient yield greater variation when done by one ophthalmologist than when done by others? We will call this the *ophthalmologist variation in replicability*.

4. Is the retinoscopic evaluation of the mean refractive error of the average person, apart from replication, essentially the same from refractionist to refractionist, or does it vary significantly?

This is not the ability of refractionists to duplicate their own readings, but rather a measure of interrefractionist variability in judgment of the magnitude of the refractive error. We will call this the *interophthalmologist variability in estimation*.

5. *Interaction*. Are some refractionists more reliable in measuring certain types of refractive error than others? Some refractionists, for example, might be more precise in measuring hyperopic errors than they would be in measuring similar degrees of myopia.

The answers to these questions might be obtained through five separate experiments, but our study was not designed that way. Such a series of experiments would have been unnecessarily difficult and time-consuming. We used a design from the area of statistics termed Analysis of Variance. This makes possible the analysis of many complex variables within a single experimental design. We present below a brief description of our sampling technique and experimental plan which resulted in an orthogonal array of data. We then present an explanation of the mathematical manipulations used to develop the analysis.

Methods

Ten subjects, five men and five women, were chosen from the secretarial, administrative, and technical staffs of the Mount Sinai Hospital. Their availability to the refractionists was one of the important requirements for selection as subjects, important because each person was examined ten different times according to a strict schedule. The subjects ranged in age from 18 to 40 years and had various forms and degrees of small refractive errors. None of the subjects had a refractive error of more than 3.00 D in any meridian, or an astigmatism larger than 2.00 D. We avoided high degrees of refractive error because we believed that they would introduce serious bias due to the chance of recognition of subjects by examiners and because we wanted to concentrate on refractive errors generally representative of the population at large. We did strive, however, to have, in our sample, equal numbers of myopes and hyperopes. An ophthalmologist, not one of the examiners in the experiment, did the initial screening and selection of the subjects.

Five ophthalmologists of varying ages and training backgrounds participated in this study.

All examinations were performed in a 20-foot room with the patient seated in an examining chair and covered from head to toe with black drapes. An ophthalmic assistant was employed to schedule the appointments, summon the patients, and arrange them in the room. When the patient had been seated in the chair completely draped, the ophthalmic assistant placed before the subject's eyes a refracting head (Greens', Bausch & Lomb) arranged with a backing of black cardboards and cloths so that no part of the subject was visible to the refractionist except the eyes as seen through the lens apertures of the refracting head. The room illumination was reduced to a standard dim level, and the ophthalmologist was then summoned. The appointments were randomized so that no ophthalmologist knew which patient he was examining. The ophthalmologists were given the freedom to choose whatever instrument they preferred and whatever method of retinoscopy with which they were most skillful. In all cases the ophthalmologists used streak retinoscopy and the method combining spheres and cylinders rather than spheres alone for their retinoscopic correcting lenses. Each patient was instructed to make no sound during the period of the retinoscopy. Following their usual practice, the ophthalmologists retinoscoped first the right and then the left eye with the patient fixating on a projected spot of light 16 feet distant from him. When his retinoscopy was completed the ophthalmologist recorded, on a printed form, the values for sphere, cylinder, and axis. After this record had been made, the subject was requested to read with this prescription from a projected chart of Snellen optotyes, and his visual acuity was recorded. The ophthalmic assistant, using a stopwatch, recorded the time spent in each phase of the examination.

Each subject was initially examined by each of the five ophthalmologists in the study. After an interval of from one to three weeks, the examinations were repeated in order to get a measure of replication under nearly identical conditions for each combination of patient and ophthalmologist. Because the subjects were well disguised and the examinations were separated in time, we can assume that the examiners did not recognize the patients or recall their refractive characteristics. Questioning of the ophthalmologists supported this assumption. In addition, we tried to prevent patient fatigue by arranging appointments so that no patient was examined by more than two ophthalmologists in succession. This plan allowed us to arrange the data in the array shown in Fig 1.

We have arranged the data in the rectangular fashion of a matrix. Each of the ophthalmologists is represented by a capital letter, A through E across the top row. The subjects are represented by the Arabic numbers that go from 1 through 10 and are arranged vertically down the left-hand column. Therefore, each cell, formed by the intersection of a column and row, represents the occasions that a specific ophthalmologist examined a specific subject. In addition, this specific subject-ophthalmologist examination occurred twice. The second subletter of the cell designation refers to either the first or the second replication. Thus, for example $C_{3,1}$ refers to ophthalmologist C examining patient 3 for the first time. $C_{3,2}$ is a similar examination done somewhat later, and for the second time.

A measure of the ability of a specific ophthalmologist to replicate his retinoscopy is given by the difference between the two measurements in each cell, eg, $C_{3,1}-C_{3,2}$. This difference may be termed d. Since this will vary from cell to cell, we give it the designation of d_i. Squaring each of these differences is convenient statistically, and we designate this new variable as $d_i{}^2$, which is directly related to the replication error.

The general measure of replication error is approximated by adding $d_i{}^2$ from all cells. Symbolically it is given in the lower right corner as $\Sigma\Sigma d^2$, the double sum of d^2 (this refers to question 1). If we add up all the $d_i{}^2$ across the columns, $\overset{\text{across columns}}{\Sigma d_i{}^2}$, each horizontal total is a measure of the "average" ophthalmologist's replication ability for each subject, the subject variability of replication. If the individual characteristics of a subject did not influence the ophthalmologists' ability to replicate his measurements, the row sums, $\overset{\text{across columns}}{\Sigma d_i{}^2}$, would be approximately equal. One of the tests we perform is the statistical evaluation of this measure of inequality (this refers to question 2). Similarly, summing the $d_i{}^2$ vertically, $\overset{\text{across rows}}{\Sigma d_i{}^2}$ (forming the column totals), yields a measure of the variability of the joint experiences of patients with individual ophthalmologists, the ophthalmologist variability in replicability. If ophthalmologists tended to have an equal replication ability, these column total replication terms would be approximately equal (this refers to question 3).

Similar manipulations of the means of the replications in each cell give us a measure of the fourth point previously mentioned: whether or not ophthalmologists generally agree in their measurement of the "average" patient, or whether there is a significant variation in preci-

20

STUDIES IN REFRACTION—SAFIR ET AL

OPHTHALMOLOGISTS

		A	B	C	D	E	AV VALUE OF ROW	COLUMNS Σd^2
	1	$A_{1,1}$ $A_{1,2}$	$B_{1,1}$ $B_{1,2}$	$C_{1,1}$ $C_{1,2}$	$D_{1,1}$ $D_{1,2}$	$E_{1,1}$ $E_{1,2}$	$\bar{X}_1$	Σd_1^2
	2		$B_{2,1}$ $B_{2,2}$				$\bar{X}_2$	Σd_2^2
	3			$C_{3,1}$ $C_{3,2}$			$\bar{X}_3$	Σd_3^2
	4				$D_{4,1}$ $D_{4,2}$			
	5					$E_{5,1}$ $E_{5,2}$		
SUBJECTS	6	$A_{6,1}$ $A_{6,2}$						
	7		$B_{7,1}$ $B_{7,2}$					
	8			$C_{8,1}$ $C_{8,2}$				
	9				$D_{9,1}$ $D_{9,2}$			
	10	$A_{10,1}$ $A_{10,2}$	$B_{10,1}$ $B_{10,2}$	$C_{10,1}$ $C_{10,2}$	$D_{10,1}$ $D_{10,2}$	$E_{10,1}$ $E_{10,2}$	$\bar{X}_{10}$	Σd_{10}^2
	AV VALUE OF COLUMN	$\bar{X}_A$	$\bar{X}_B$			$\bar{X}_E$	$\bar{\bar{X}}$ = GRAND AV	
	ROWS Σd^2	d_A^2	d_B^2			d_E^2	ROW Σ	COLUMN Σd^2

Fig 1.—Data array for any one variable.

sion, or lack of agreement in their judgment. If we average the means from all the cells in a column, $\bar{X}_a$ $\bar{X}_b$, . . . $\bar{X}_e$, each average represents the specific ophthalmologist's judgment of the refractive error of the average subject who is a composite of the ten different subjects. If ophthalmologists tend to agree in their mea-

surements, there will be little difference in these averages. We test the nature of these differences statistically and judge whether or not they are significantly different from zero (this refers to question 4).

Finally the interaction term is statistically evaluated (this refers to question 5).

21

OPHTHALMOLOGISTS

		A	B	C	D	E	ROW MEAN	SUM OF VARI-ANCES
1	MEAN	0.6250	0.3750	0.6250	0.2500	0	0.3750	
	VARIANCE	0.0312	0.0312	0.0313	0.1250	0		0.2186
2	MEAN	−1.0000	−1.3750	−1.2500	−1.2500	−1.2500	−1.2250	
	VARIANCE	0.1250	0.0312	0.1250	0	0		0.2812
3	MEAN	−2.7500	−1.6250	−2.1250	−1.8750	−1.8750	−2.0500	
	VARIANCE	0	0.0312	0.0312	0.0312	0.0312		0.1248
4	MEAN	1.0000	1.2500	0.8750	1.1250	1.0000	1.0500	
	VARIANCE	0.5000	0	0.0312	0.0312	0		0.5624
5	MEAN	−0.2500	0	−0.2500	0	0.1250	−0.0750	
	VARIANCE	0.1250	0	0	0	0.0312		0.1562
6	MEAN	−1.6250	−1.5000	−1.6250	−2.0000	−1.5000	−1.6500	
	VARIANCE	0.0312	0.1250	0.0312	0.1250	0		0.3124
7	MEAN	0	0.2500	−0.2500	0	0.5000	0.1000	
	VARIANCE	0.5000	0	0.1250	0	0		0.6250
8	MEAN	0.7500	0.3750	0.5000	−0.2500	0.1250	0.3000	
	VARIANCE	0.1250	0.0312	0.1250	0.1250	0.0312		0.4374
9	MEAN	−1.8750	−2.3750	−2.0000	−2.6250	−2.2500	−2.2250	
	VARIANCE	0.7812	0.0312	0.5000	0.0312	0.1250		1.4686
10	MEAN	−3.0000	−3.0000	−2.8750	−2.8750	−2.6250	−2.8750	
	VARIANCE	0	0	0.0312	0.0312	0.0312		0.0936
	COLUMN MEAN	−0.8125	−0.7625	−0.8375	−0.9500	−0.7750	−0.8275 GRAND MEAN	
	SUM OF VARIANCES	2.2186	0.2810	1.0310	0.4998	0.2498	TOTAL VARIATION 4.2802	

SUBJECTS

Fig 2.—Sphere, right eye.

Two-way analyses of variance with replication were performed with the aid of a computer (IBM 360-67). A separate analysis was performed with respect to each of the following variables: sphere power, cylinder power, left or right eye, male, or female. This generated eight matrices such as that shown in Fig 1. The data presented below are given in a matrix form, but within each cell of the matrix are given the mean and variance of the two measurements. The variance (the square of the SD) is directly proportional to the Σd_i^2 previously described. Because of space limitations, the individual measurements are not given, but the interested reader may readily calculate them from the data supplied.

Unless otherwise stated, all tests of significance were carried out at a significance level of 5%.

Results

Male-Female Differences.—No significant differences were found in respect to the variables measured; we were therefore able to fuse the data from all ten subjects for subsequent analyses.

Sphere-Right Eye.—The summary data are given in Fig 2 and the analysis of variance in Table 1.

1. A measure of the general replicability is given by the square root of the within-

Table 1.—*Analysis of Variance*

Source of Variation	Degrees of Freedom	Sum of Squares	Mean Square	F
Ophthalmologists (O)	4	0.446	0.111	0.770
Patients (P)	9	161.431	17.937	209.540
O×P (interaction)	36	5.181	0.144	1.681
Within replications	50	4.280	0.086	...
Total	99	175.832	...	...

mean-square, 0.086. This value, the standard deviation, equals 0.293 D. In clinical terms, we can state that it is highly improbable that any two replicate retinoscopy measurements of sphere power made by the "average" ophthalmologist on the "average" subject will differ from each other by more than 1.34 D. (This estimate was derived from the concept of tolerance limits. We chose to include 95% of the population with 90% confidence.) Put in other terms, if the average ophthalmologist makes two separate retinoscopic measurements of sphere power on the same subject, and these measurements differ from each other by less than 1.34 D, you *may not* state that the chances are as good as 9 out of 10 that the two measurements are truly different.

2. The subject variability of replication shows considerable differences among patients. For example, the average variability of the ophthalmologists' measurement of subject 9 was more than ten times greater than the variability in measurement of subject 10. However, when Bartlett's test for the homogeneity of variance was used to evaluate the meaning of these differences among all ten subjects, the differences were found to be of only borderline significance.

3. Ophthalmologists do differ significantly in their ability to replicate measurements on the various patients. For example, ophthalmologist A shows nearly ten times the variability of ophthalmologists B or E.

4. Ophthalmologists do not differ significantly in their evaluation of the mean spherical error for the right eye of the average patient. Examination of the column means of Fig 2 demonstrates this.

5. There is no significant interaction effect.

Sphere—Left Eye (Fig 3 and Table 2). —1. The ability of the "average" ophthalmologist to replicate his own measurements is not significantly different in the left eye as compared to the right.

2. As in the case of the right eye, there are only borderline differences in replication error for different subjects.

3. As in the case of the right eye, there is significant variation among ophthalmologists in their ability to replicate measurements of various individuals.

There is great internal consistency among the examiners in the relative magnitude of these abilities to replicate. For example, ophthalmologist A shows the greatest variability, C the next to greatest, and E the least in both right and left eyes.

In addition, the absolute magnitudes of these variations are always greater in the left eye than in the right.

4. In contrast to the findings on the right eye, ophthalmologists do differ significantly in their evaluation of the mean spherical error of the left eye of the average patient.

5. There was no significant interaction.

Cylinder Power—Right Eye (Fig 4 and Table 3). —1. The within-mean square equals 0.056. Its square root, the standard deviation, equals 0.237. Thus, it is very improbable that any two replicate measurements of cylinder power made on the same subject will differ by more than 1.08 D.

2. The subject variability of replication shows no significant or borderline difference.

3. There are no significant differences in the abilities of the various ophthalmologists to replicate their measurements of the various subjects.

4. There was no significant interophthalmologist variation in estimation of the mean cylinder power, right eye.

5. There was no significant interaction.

Cylinder Power—Left Eye (Fig 5 and Table 4). —1. The within-mean-square equals

www.ingramcontent.com/pod-product-compliance
Lightning Source LLC
Chambersburg PA
CBHW080631180526
45168CB00007B/3122